1

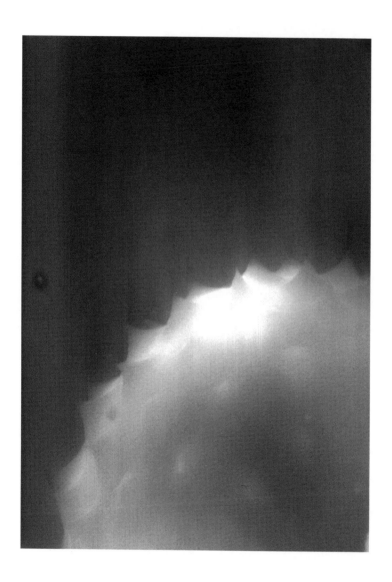

THE SECRETS OF SARS-CoV-2

By Carlo Brogna

The research about the SARS-CoV-2 bacteriophage, the bacteria it interacts with, and the world of toxins.

The images no one has shown you before.

Cover image:

SEM image. HV 20.00kV, curr 0,33nA, mag 15000, aperture 50µ. A part of SARS-CoV-2 in a faecal sample during the seven-day microbiological culture. -

Author: Carlo Brogna

- Director and scientific coordinator at Craniomed Group, Italy;
- Doctor of Medicine and Surgery (The University of Salerno, Italy);
- Doctor of Dental Medicine and Prosthodontist (Gabriele d'Annunzio University of Chieti, Italy);
- Specialist orthodontist (Gabriele d'Annunzio University of Chieti, Italy);
- Master of Science in gnathology and orofacial pain (Gabriele d'Annunzio University of Chieti, Italy);
- Continuing dental education program in oral surgery (NJDS, USA);
- Collaborator and scientific support specialist at one of the leading companies specialized in dental implants and bone biomaterials (TBR Group, France);
- Experienced in maxillofacial and oral surgery (University "Renè Descartes", France).

"Imagination is more important than knowledge. For knowledge is limited, whereas imagination embraces the entire world, stimulating progress, giving birth to evolution."

Albert Einstein - Interview by George Sylvester Viereck

The Saturday Evening Post (26 October 1929).

CONTENTS

Part 3

Part 4

Part 1

Foreword

In January 1610, Galileo Galilei observed four celestial bodies similar to stars near the planet Jupiter, using a telescope of his manufacture, not even certified yet (the certificate of conformity was issued on 22nd July 1993).

Two-month night work, unpaid and uninsured, led to the discovery of Medici Stars (Io, Europa, Ganymede, and Callisto), the "stars" that revolve around Jupiter.

Thanks to scientific development, we know that what the Pisan called "stars" are actually the Galilean moons, and their exact number is 79, not 4.

Fortunately, Galileo did not receive a Nobel Prize or even a doctorate. Thus, he managed to avoid spending a significant amount of his time on webinars and meetings, articles, publishing, and double (if not triple) judging. Galileo wrote a simple book, illustrated by hand, with no bibliography, to share his observations with everyone (Galileo Galilei, Sidereus Nuncius - Il Messaggero Delle Stelle, 1610).

Yet, every self-respecting scientist in the world knows what the Galilean Method is.

Well, dear reader, whether you are a qualified academic researcher or an ordinary human being, you should know - what

I propose is a result of intuitive actions, simple tests, and observations.

I have mentioned the great astronomer because I am trying to inspire you to improve and enhance the new approach to the study of SARS-CoV-2.

With all my respect for this historical figure, I am not trying to compare myself to him in any way.

Carlo Brogna

Methodology

The images, presented in this volume, were taken during the *microscopic* examination of SARS-CoV-2 infected *faecal samples* collected for culture. Viral replication was monitored using Luminex-technology on days 7, 14, and 30 (NxTAG®CoV Extended Panel, a real-time reverse transcriptase PCR assay detecting three SARS-CoV-2 genes was used on the MAGPIX®NxTAG-enabled System MAGPIX instrument). The signal acquisition was performed using the xPONENT and SYNCT software, Luminex Molecular Diagnostic.

The culture was performed using the "Brogna-Petrillo" method described in the scientific paper *"Petrillo and Others, 'Increase of SARS-CoV-2 RNA Load in Faecal Samples Prompts for Rethinking of SARS-CoV-2 Biology and COVID-19 Epidemiology', 2020 https://doi.org/10.5281/zenodo.4088208"*.

Image quality:

SEM: samples were observed at 20 kV, using either backscattered electrons (BSE) or secondary electrons (SE); FIB-SEM (FEI Versa 3D model) uses a field emission gun (FEG).

TEM - FEI Tecnai F20 with FEG source. Most of the images were taken at 120kV and only a few at 200kV. All the images were acquired in the bright field mode with an objective aperture between 60 and 100. Some pictures are slightly out of focus to help visualize details.

The samples were prepared using osmium tetroxide.

Introduction

SARS-CoV-2 and the coronavirus infection caused by it bring new challenges for the Global Scientific Community. This is a battle yet to be won. For now, it continues to affect our everyday life.

Instead of waiting for a solution, like manna from heaven, every person should contribute to the common good.

The scientists give their contribution, combining their work with study, research and experimentation. While the majority, should try obtaining the correct information and defending the ideas that do not have any influential support or popularity amongst the media sources. It is important to reinforce sound ideas, even before they are proven true and decisive in the evolutionary process. Only this way, we can be sure that our fate will not depend on elective decisions.

We cannot afford the luxury of leaving some ideas unnoticed. History of science and world history *docent*.

You often end up hitting a rubber wall trying to bring your scientific evidence to the attention of an influential audience.

Further, we would like to talk about certain scientific evidence, and we will try to keep it short and simple, wherever possible.

When the coronaviruses were first described in 1951, they were classified as microorganisms capable of infecting epithelial cells, like the ones that our skin, mucous membranes, lungs, and liver are composed of.

Until a few months ago, we were still anchored to that discovery.

Since then, in fact, no one has ever wondered if coronaviruses are capable of infecting only and exclusively the epithelial cells. No one has ever proved, nor denied, whether this virus family has other targets as well.

The crux of the new horizon we are about to present is that our scientific study shows SARS-CoV-2 while infecting other cell types.

We are certain that SARS-CoV-2 is also a bacteriophage, meaning that it is capable of infecting bacteria. We can also provide visual evidence to prove this fact. Our research results show that this virus infects bacteria within human gut microbiota (Fig. 1-2).

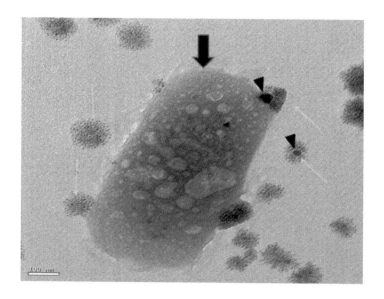

Figure 1: TEM image. An unidentified bacterium (big arrow) and SARS-CoV-2 (arrowheads) in a faecal sample during the seven-day culture. Thin arrows indicate the toxins/proteins. Dr C. Brogna - Craniomed Group. All rights reserved.

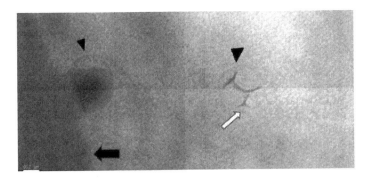

Figure 2: TEM image. A faecal sample during the seven-day culture. SARS-CoV-2 and the bacterial cell wall. There is the virus (arrowhead) interacting with the bacterium (big arrow). The image also shows a virus (arrowhead) without its RNA; there is just a mysterious "endoskeleton" left inside it (white arrow). Dr C. Brogna - Craniomed Group. All rights reserved.

In this image, it seems that the virus (a dark particle on the left) is inoculating its genetic content using a typical bacteriophage mechanism.

This event triggers a series of microbiological and biochemical events, with consequent clinical implications, which no one has ever considered before.

Nevertheless, all efforts to end this pandemic continue focusing on the outdated image of the virus and bacteria.

However, it is rather clear that the coronaviruses are a quite peculiar virus family:

17

- In the late 1990s, Dr Sawicki of the University of Toledo (Ohio, USA) described an abnormal way coronavirus replicate. They read and replicate RNA filaments using a "jump" model, at 3'-5'.[1]

- Dr Clark describes a possibility that coronaviruses may contain the genetic information, necessary to synthesize conotoxins.[2]

- In 2000, Fernando Almazán, Silvia Márquez-Jurado, Aitor Nogales, and Luis Enjuanes learned how to replicate transmissible gastroenteritis coronavirus (TGEV) in pigs using a bacterial artificial plasmid. These authors' latest studies confirm that this method is also applicable to the coronavirus MERS (Middle East Respiratory Stress Syndrome - 2012/2013) study. It is possible to place the genomic sequence of this coronavirus into a bacterial artificial plasmid Escherichia Coli (bacterial artificial chromosome or BAC), adding Cytomegalovirus promoter sequences and hepatitis D virus sequences in order to examine it better.

---

[1]Sawicki, S. G. and D. L. Sawicki, 'A New Model for Coronavirus Transcription', *Advances in Experimental Medicine and Biology,* 440 (1998), 215–19 <https://doi.org/10.1007/978-1-4615-5331-1_26>. Sawicki, S. G. and D. L. Sawicki, 'A New Model for Coronavirus Transcription', *Advances in Experimental Medicine and Biology,* 440 (1998), 215–19 <https://doi.org/10.1007/978-1-4615-5331-1_26>.
[2] *Biotechnology*, 2nd edition (Academic Cell, 2015).

Laboratories studying SARS-CoV-2 analyse the virus's interactions with synthetic cells ("Vero Cell" and such)[3] in a decontaminated working environment, where, according to the protocol, to eliminate bacteria, they use antibiotics. Similar circumstances "might" affect virus activity, and this is the main mistake. Eliminating important "actors" from the virus development cycle might trigger its aggression. It is the same as saying that a human being lacks the ability to survive on Earth while observing him or her on a tiny desert island, "in a company" of a sole coconut palm. In such conditions, we know that very few individuals would survive, and surely, no one would be able to build a hut. However, if the same individual were to enter a different context - a larger island with a greater variety and quantity of fruit plants, he would have a higher chance of survival. Moreover, this human would have the possibility to apply his or her creativity and manual skills to build shelter and procure food. The exclusive study of SARS-CoV-2 in a "Vero Cell", similar to the human eukaryotic cell but still not identical to it, is limiting and limited. It does not allow contemplating other possible biological and biochemical interactions that the virus can establish with other types of cells, like the ones I observed between SARS-CoV-2 and bacteria within the human gut microbiota. Koch's second postulate (1843–1910) states: "The pathogen can be isolated from the diseased host and grown in *pure culture*". This statement could

[3] Nicole C. Ammerman, Magda Beier-Sexton, and Abdu F. Azad, 'Growth and Maintenance of Vero Cell Lines', *Current Protocols in Microbiology*, APPENDIX (2008), Appendix-4E <https://doi.org/10.1002/9780471729259.mca04es11>.

be applicable for a disease like tuberculosis, but in our case, it should be rephrased:

"A pathogen must be observed in both - pure culture and mixed environment, together with other microorganisms, in order to analyse its interactions with other species, as well as its individual characteristics".

Experiments

One of the most frequent symptoms of COVID-19 is the loss of smell (hyposmia). Intrigued by the fact that it was observed only in 1/3 part of all the cases, we began investigating all the possible causes of this clinical manifestation, heterogeneously distributed among the infected symptomatic population.

We have evaluated two possible causes of smell reduction.

1. SARS-CoV-2 infects neurons of the olfactory bulb, causing inflammatory alterations that undermine its proper functioning, which subsequently prevents the odour "collection".

2. Odour collection occurs normally, but the information transmission is blocked along the way by a neurotransmitter called **acetylcholine.** Consequently, this information never reaches the temporal cerebral cortex, where the "smell" is recognised on a conscious level.

To investigate the second possibility more thoroughly, we needed to establish what compromised the functions of acetylcholine.

To this end, we analysed the RNA genome of SARS-CoV-2, made available by our Chinese colleagues. During the research, we noticed that after infecting a cell, the virus is able to program

21

it to synthesise proteins, similar to toxins produced by some poisonous animals.[4]

In other words, it was clear that the virus has a recipe for the production of these toxic substances. However, it is not determined yet whether the virus can obtain all the necessary ingredients and tools to "finish the production".

Further, we inspected the plasma and urine specimens of COVID-19 patients for this kind of proteins.

Subjecting all the participants' plasma and urine specimens to mass spectrometry, we isolated more than 80 proteins, exerting various biological effects. These proteins, however, turned out to be absent in plasma and urine of healthy patients. It means that the virus was able to process the recipe (fig.3-5).[5]

[4]Carlo Brogna, 'The COVID-19 Virus Double Pathogenic Mechanism. A New Perspective', 2020 <https://doi.org/10.20944/preprints202004.0165.v2>.

[5] Carlo Brogna and others, 'Detection of Toxin-like Peptides in Plasma and Urine Samples from COVID-19 Patients', 2020 <https://doi.org/10.5281/zenodo.4139341>.

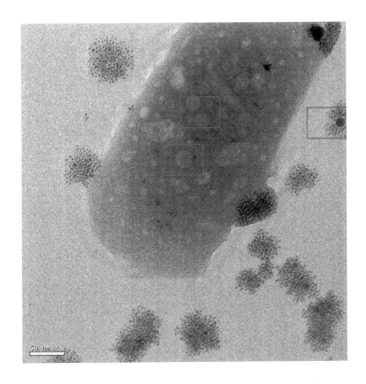

Figure 3: TEM image. A faecal sample during the seven-day culture. SARS-CoV-2 is visible in the rectangular area. Dr C. Brogna - Craniomed Group.

Amongst the proteins obtained from the bacterial-viral interaction, there were **several forms of conotoxins** (powerful neurotoxins already known to be the chemical weapon used by conical snails to capture their prey). Some of these conotoxins were able to occupy and block the acetylcholine binding sites (binding of acetylcholine allows to transmit olfactory information to the brain).

Finally, it became clear; we understood the pattern of hyposmia and how it manifests itself in the symptomatic individuals. The last thing to discover was why not all the COVID-19 patients presented this symptom.

The answer was hidden in the variety of conotoxins found — these molecules are very similar to each other, but they have slightly different structural details.

Comparing various forms of conotoxins, we found that some of them have only slight differences between their amino acid sequences. This observation suggested that their existence was conditioned by "assembly errors". Because of these mistakes, the molecules were produced with small "factory defects", nonconforming according to the initial "project", i.e., the recipe of SARS-CoV-2 RNA.

These "factory defects" are typical for the synthesis of proteins in bacteria - a much more tumultuous, rapid and imprecise process, than the one that characterises eukaryotic cells (human epithelial cells, for example). Therefore, we decided to investigate whether bacterial and not epithelial cells produced these toxins.

The hypothesis was that SARS-CoV-2 uses gut bacteria to produce the toxins we found in the plasma and urine specimens of COVID-19 patients. To validate this assumption, we needed

24

to document that the virus is capable of infecting prokaryotic cells, such as bacteria. Since 1951, no one has ever doubted that coronaviruses infect only epithelial cells.

For this purpose, the faeces of healthy patients were inoculated with SARS-CoV-2. Shortly, we received confirmation that the virus is replicating inside the faeces. Meaning that the faeces, or bacteria present in healthy patients' faeces, to be precise, are fertile ground for viral replication. All the process is captured in photographs.[6]

In medical terms, SARS-CoV-2 can **also be classified as a bacteriophage** (Fig. 3, 4-6) - a virus capable of infecting bacteria and replicating within them, contemporarily stimulating the synthesis of their proteins. Because of the hectic bacterial metabolic activity, this process does not always end perfectly and accordingly to the initial "project". In fact, some of the proteins, produced by gut bacteria on the virus orders, end up being malfunctioning, in the case with conotoxins - unable to block acetylcholine.

Therefore, hyposmia occurs only in patients, whose gut bacteria produce a significant amount of normally formed and functioning conotoxins that occupy acetylcholine receptors, freezing the transmission of a nerve impulse along the olfactory pathways.

---

[6] Mauro Petrillo and others, 'Increase of SARS-CoV-2 RNA Load in Faecal Samples Prompts for Rethinking of SARS-CoV-2 Biology and COVID-19 Epidemiology', 2020 <https://doi.org/10.5281/zenodo.4088208>.

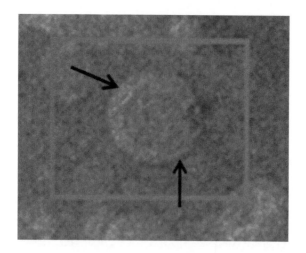

Figure 4 (3): TEM image. A faecal sample during the seven-day culture. In the rectangular area – SARS-CoV-2 inside the bacterium. You can also see the "corona" of the virus (black arrow). Dr C. Brogna - Craniomed Group.

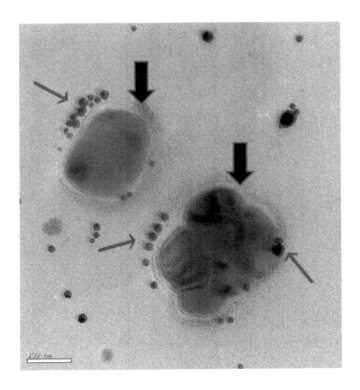

Figure 5: TEM image. A faecal sample during the seven-day culture. SARS-CoV-2 and the bacteria (mycoplasma?). The virus (thin arrows) is interacting with the bacteria (big arrow). Dr C. Brogna - Craniomed Group. All rights reserved.

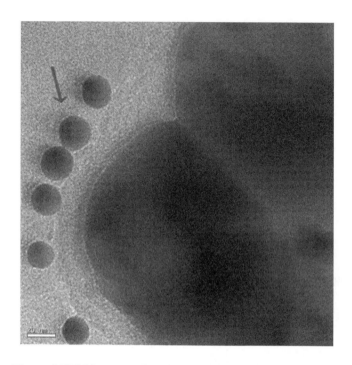

Figure 6: TEM image. A faecal sample during the seven-day culture. SARS-CoV-2 and the bacterium, enlarged detail from Figure 5. Dr C. Brogna - Craniomed Group. All rights reserved.

Analysis

There is a good possibility that the symptoms of COVID-19 are caused by some kind of "poisoning".

This may be too rash, but the fact is that proteins, similar to those found in the animal venoms, have been found in the plasma and urine samples of all symptomatic patients tested. At the same time, the proteins of this kind were absent in the healthy patients' specimens.

Once infected with SARS-CoV-2, gut bacteria start synthesising proteins with toxin-like activity, primarily:

- **Conotoxins:** potent neurotoxins produced by cone snails that live in tropical and subtropical seas. These toxins can increase the activity of the parasympathetic nervous system on a par with drugs designed especially for this purpose (antihypertensive drugs, for example).

- **Phospholipase A2:** a protein that triggers a biochemical cascade, causing excessive blood clotting (Thromboxane A2) and bronchoconstriction (Leukotrienes). These effects are enhanced by taking common anti-inflammatory drugs (acetylsalicylic acid, ibuprofen, etc.).

- **Prothrombin** activator: a protein that stimulates the last stage of the blood coagulation cascade. Accelerated

29

coagulation creates microemboli. Many experts in the field report that this phenomenon is often observed in patients infected with COVID-19.

- **Many other proteins, such as** phosphodiesterase, zinc metalloproteinase, serine protease, bradykinin, etc. (for more information, see C. Brogna and others, 'Detection of Toxin-like Peptides in Plasma and Urine Samples from COVID-19 Patients', 2020 <https://doi.org/10.5281/zenodo.4139341).

Knowing how exactly the virus manages to infect the gut bacteria and enlist them for the production of toxin-like products, we could find a way to treat the symptoms of the disease directly. This is as important as having an effective vaccine. Besides, this solution might be even cheaper and easier to achieve.

Discovering the dominant role of gut bacteria in viral replication changes therapeutic and epidemiological approaches to the disease. The actions should be taken immediately, right from the moment SARS-CoV-2 particles, viable and capable of infecting, are found in the patient's faeces.

This means that the patients declared healthy after performing a nasopharyngeal swab remain contagious. People around them can still be infected via the faecal-oral route or by touching the infected surfaces.

The negative result of a nasal swab does not exclude the contagiousness, considering that the virus may also have its own occult gastrointestinal reserve.

Moreover, these findings suggest that the bacteria engineer the virus, creating many **mutations** in it. This process is called **"Editing"** (CRISP model). The gut bacteria perform such actions to protect themselves from a future[7] attack, but, unfortunately, they generate chaos in the host's body along the way. These consequences leave room for all kinds of scenarios.

[7]Rodolphe Barrangou and others, 'CRISPR Provides Acquired Resistance against Viruses in Prokaryotes', *Science (New York, N.Y.)* , 315.5819 (2007), 1709–12 <https://doi.org/10.1126/science.1138140>.

Discussion

Having an effective COVID-19 vaccine at your disposal already is or could be a great achievement. However, it is difficult to create a reliable "protective shield" without knowing the nature of the threat and its mechanisms. We cannot declare the end of the war yet, because, sometimes, shields also have "factory defects".

For this reason, the discoveries illustrated so far, and the therapeutic aspects that accompany them may be as important as the development of an effective vaccine.

Having a **plan B** is much more reassuring, especially if the shield were to malfunction.

After carrying out these experiments, we can sum up that:

- First of all, the disease should be treated as a **poisoning syndrome.** Then, the toxins, causing the symptoms of COVID-19, should be neutralised using **antidotes.** Only hyper-specialised laboratories have means for decoding the toxic protein structure and synthesising the bespoken antidotes, which "adapt" and deactivate these toxins.

- In addition to the antidotes that inactivate already produced and circulating toxins, it is important to stop the

32

production of new toxins. In other words, it is necessary to temporarily "freeze" the gut bacteria, which, affected by SARS-CoV-2, synthesise toxic proteins, using **bacteriostatic or bactericidal** drugs. The early administration of azithromycin, vancomycin, or metronidazole allows preventing viral replication and toxin synthesis (in vitro) Amoxicillin, on the other hand, while blocking viral replication, does not stop the toxin production completely. Along with antibiotic therapy, probiotics should be used as **adjuvant therapy.**

- The positive clinical effects of antibiotic therapy (usually not indicated for the treatment of a viral infection) confirm the central role of gut bacteria in the genesis of clinical manifestations of COVID-19. Similarly, empirical use of **dexamethasone** was found useful in containing the symptoms of COVID-19. This drug inhibits Phospholipase A2 - one of the toxin-like proteins found in infected patients, notorious for its capability to activate a cascade of biochemical events underlying the clinical picture of COVID-19.

- In cases with symptomatic COVID-19 patients whose general state of health is already compromised (individuals with concomitant cardiovascular diseases, for example), it is necessary to avoid the administration of drugs that could precipitate their primary pathological condition (cardiac pathology, in the present case). The administration of cycloxygenase-1 (COX-1) inhibitors, i.e., acetylsalicylic acid, ibuprofen, etc., is to be avoided because it enhances the production of:

-Thromboxane; it causes vasoconstriction and platelet aggregation that could dramatically worsen the clinical picture of symptomatic COVID+ patients with cardiovascular disorders.

-Leukotrienes; excessive lipoxygenase activity causes the bronchoconstriction, which can undoubtedly lead to a fatal outcome of patients with concomitant diseases of the respiratory tree.

PART 2

Toxins

As previously mentioned, there is a real possibility that a certain kind of "poisoning" causes the symptoms of COVID-19. Toxin-like proteins were found in the plasma and urine samples from all the symptomatic patients examined. Once infected with the bacteriophage SARS-CoV-2, gut microbiota starts synthesising proteins, similar to those found in some animal poisons.

Amongst the many toxin-like proteins found (Fig. 7-12), the ones of greatest interest are:

- conotoxins;
- phospholipase A2;
- prothrombin-activator;
- many other proteins, such as phosphodiesterase, zinc metalloproteinase, serine protease, bradykinin, etc. (for more information, see C. Brogna and others, 'Detection of Toxin-like Peptides in Plasma and Urine Samples from COVID-19 Patients', 2020 <https://doi.org/10.5281/zenodo.4139341).[8]

---

[8] Brogna and others. 'Detection of Toxin-like Peptides in Plasma and Urine Samples from COVID-19 Patients', 2020 <https://doi.org/10.5281/zenodo.4139341>.

Conotoxins

Conotoxins - potent neurotoxins produced by conical snails living in tropical and subtropical areas. These peptides increase the activity of the parasympathetic nervous system because of their link with cholinesterase. Different conotoxin-cholinesterase complexes can have various biological activities. Regardless of all this, we can say that the dysfunction of the cholinergic system plays a key role in the pathogenesis of clinical manifestations of COVID-19.

Acetylcholine (ACh) is one of the best-characterised neurotransmitters. It plays a central role in cholinergic synapses of the central and peripheral (PNS) nervous system (CNS). ACh was the first molecule identified as a neurotransmitter and appears to be one of the phylogenetically oldest signalling molecules. In fact, it has been detected in bacteria, protozoa, fungi, algae, and primitive plants, proving that the living organisms had a cholinergic system before it appeared in the nervous system. The autonomic nervous system (ANS) is an integral part of natural history. It triggers the fight-or-flight response and regulates the biological rhythms of all vital and cognitive functions. Therefore, observing hyposmia or dysgeusia in COVID-19 patients was like getting lucky on a bad day. It allowed us to understand the situation better and hypothesise that something was wrong with their autonomic nervous system and that the cholinergic system was involved. Other researchers had similar observations as well.[9,10]

[9] 'The Role of Nicotine in COVID-19 Infection', *The Centre for Evidence-Based Medicine* <https://www.cebm.net/covid-19/nicotine-replacement-therapy/> [accessed 27 December 2020].
[10] 'COVID-19 and Smoking: Is Nicotine the Hidden Link? | European Respiratory Society' <https://erj.ersjournals.com/content/55/6/2001116> [accessed 27 December 2020].

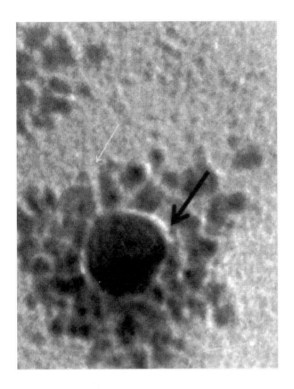

Figure 7: TEM image. SARS-CoV-2 in a faecal sample during the seven-day culture. You can see its "corona" (black arrow) and the proteins/toxins (thin arrows) around it. Dr C. Brogna - Craniomed Group. All rights reserved.

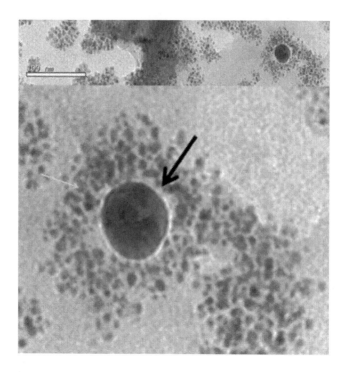

Figure 8: TEM image. A faecal sample during the seven-day culture. An enlarged photo of SARS-CoV-2. You can see its "corona" (black arrow) and the proteins/toxins (thin arrows) around it. Dr C. Brogna - Craniomed Group. All rights reserved.

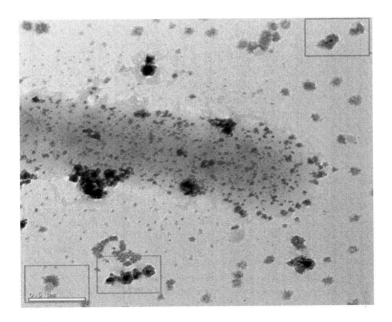

Figure 9: TEM image. A faecal sample after the seven-day culture. SARS-CoV-2 is in the rectangular area. Dr C. Brogna - Craniomed Group.

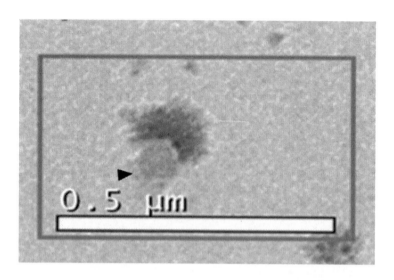

Figure 10: TEM image. SARS-CoV-2 (arrowhead) and the toxins (thin arrow) in a faecal specimen. Dr C. Brogna - Craniomed Group. All rights reserved.

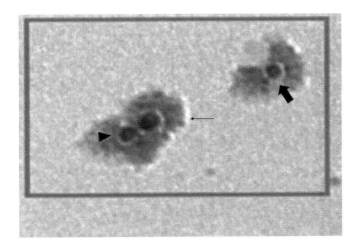

Figure 11: TEM image. SARS-CoV-2 (arrowhead) and the toxins (thin arrow) in a faecal specimen. A typical "corona" is visible around the particles of the virus (black arrow). Dr C. Brogna -

43

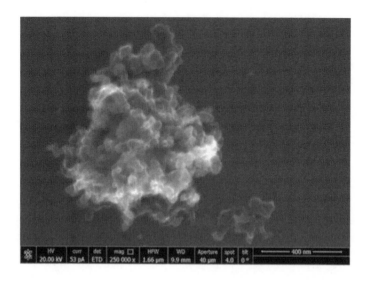

Figure 12: SEM image. An ultrastructural form of a protein/toxin in a SARS-CoV-2 contaminated faecal sample. Dr C. Brogna - Craniomed Group.

44

Cholinesterase

Cholinesterase is the target for toxins present in many animal poisons.

Toxins produced by snakes Naja Atra, Bungarus multicinctus, and Bungarus fasciatus, as well as by cone snails, inhibit the function of acetylcholinesterase, and **butyrylcholinesterase (pseudocholinesterase)** in particular. Thus, cholinesterase levels, regulating the liver function, can be used as an indirect marker of poisoning. The symptom duration is largely determined by characteristics of the toxic complex, such as liposolubility; the need for metabolic activation; stability of the toxin-AChE complex; "ageing" of the phosphorylated enzyme.[11]

The pathogenesis of toxic effects, mediated by conotoxins, or rather all molecules that hold cholinesterase acetates, depends on the acetylcholine (ACh) level and agonist activity (they are blocking nicotinic receptors). Some toxin-acetyl-cholinesterase complexes do not catalyse acetylcholine.

<In the first case, toxic manifestations are the consequence of increased acetylcholine (ACh) action *on muscarinic receptors of*

---

[11] Mr Brogna. Brogna, C. The COVID-19 Virus Double Pathogenic Mechanism. A New Perspective. Preprints 2020, 2020040165 (doi: 10.20944/preprints202004.0165.v2). Here you can find all the referencees.

45

type M2 and M3. The occupation of M2 receptors by [12] *high ACh titles* determine generalized vasodilation and consequent rapid drop in blood *pressure; bradycardia effect (slowing heart activity and reduction of heart range), followed by arrhythmic and tachycardia compensation. It should be added, however, that these manifestations can be added to changes in the rhythm related to hypoxemia - antagonized by assisted pulmonary ventilation; direct action on vasomotor centers and other cardiovascular centers of the elongated marrow, which aggravates leads to hypotension and the consequent reflex fibrillations and tachycardias'. The occupation of* M3 *muscarinic* receptors *by* high *ACh* titles *determine hypersecretion of bronchial* mucous membranes *with vasoconstriction; increased gastrointestinal motility. Some toxins also have properties like nicotinic receptor agonists: in this case, at the level of neuromuscular joints, nicotinic agonist action is manifested by muscle fatigue and general weakness; involuntary contractions and collation. In particular, asthenia, up to paralysis, of the diaphragm and intercostal muscles, combined with the muscarinic and nicotinic effects of CNS (laryngospasm, bronchoconstriction, bronchial hypersecretion, which all contribute to respiratory impairment), determine clinical manifestations ranging from the sense of constriction to the chest to dyspnea, up to prolonged apnea and respiratory depression. Other effects on the CNS are confusion, ataxia,*

---

[12] 'Goodman & Gilman's: The Pharmacological Basis of Therapeutics, 13e | AccessMedicine | McGraw-Hill Medical' <https://accessmedicine.mhmedical.com/book.aspx?bookID=2189> [accessed December 27, 2020].

verbal confusion, loss of reflexes, Cheyne-Stokes breathing, seizures, coma and respiratory paralysis. The eye symptoms, which may also be related to local exposure to toxic aerosol, are myosis, eye pain, conjunctival congestion, reduced vision, ciliary spasm and eyebrow pain. Following acute systemic absorption, however, myosis is not highlighted due to a powerful sympathetic discharge in response to hypotension. In case of high doses of toxins, the clinical picture can present violently, with extreme salivation, involuntary emission of feces and urine, sweating, tearing, bradycardia, hypotension, arrhythmias, and cardiovascular collapse. Finally, among the non-specific symptoms, which include nausea, vomiting, abdominal cramps and diarrhea, anosmia and dysgeusia should be emphasized>.[13]

Olfactory dysfunction is an early "preclinical" sign of Parkinson's disease (usually, it is the first one to appear). It often remains the only symptom until a specialist diagnoses the disease. Unfortunately, by that time, more than 80% of GABAergic neurons are usually lost.[14] It is important to remember that these neural pathways do not cross thalamic nuclei. They adhere directly to the amygdala and hippocampal complex. Nicotine binding to the receptor is substantially reduced in all disorders associated with a presynaptic cortical cholinergic deficit. For example, Alzheimer's disease,

---

[13] 'Goodman & Gilman's: The Pharmacological Basis of Therapeutics, 13e | AccessMedicine | McGraw-Hill Medical'.

[14] Michelle E. Fullard, James F. Morley, and John E. Duda, 'Olfactory Dysfunction as an Early Biomarker in Parkinson's Disease', *Neuroscience Bulletin*, 33.5 (2017), 515–25 <https://doi.org/10.1007/s12264-017-0170-x>.

Parkinson's disease and Down's syndrome are characterized by extensive loss of choline acetyltransferase. On the contrary, muscarinic receptor (M1 and M2) activity reduction is moderate in Alzheimer's disease and increased (apparently unrelated to anticholinergic medications) in Parkinson's disease in cases with dementia (but not in cases without it).[15]

[15]E.K. Perry and others, 'Cholinergic Receptors in Cognitive Disorders', *Canadian Journal of Neurological Sciences / Journal Canadien Des Sciences Neurologiques*,13.S4 (1986), 521–27 <https://doi.org/10.1017/S0317167100037240>.

Phospholipase

Phospholipase A2 (PLA2) is characterised as one of the most abundant proteins in snake venom. It is a hydrolase that performs a broad spectrum of toxic pharmacological activities.[16]

J.B. Harris et al. describe the main types of PLA2: secreted PLA2 (sPLA2); cytosolic PLA2 (cPLA2); calcium-independent PLA2 (iPLA2); platelet-activating factor (PAF); lipoprotein-associated PLA2 (LpPLA2); adipose PLA2 (AdPLA2s); lysosomal PLA2 (LPLA2s). PLA2 triggers the inflammatory response by stimulating the release of mediators such as IL-1β, IL-6, IL-8, TNF-α, MIP-1α, NO, histamine, serotonin, PAF, bradykinin, PGE2, TXA2, LTB4, RANTES, and anaphylaxis (C3 and C5).[17] By mediating the hydrolysis of glycerophospholipids, PLA2 determines the release of fatty acids and the related production of lysophospholipids.[18]

---

[16] Raoudha Zouari-Kessentini and others, 'Antitumoral Potential of Tunisian Snake Venoms Secreted Phospholipases A2', *BioMed Research International*, 2013 (2013) <https://doi.org/10.1155/2013/391389>.

[17] Catarina Teixeira and others, 'Inflammation Induced by Platelet-Activating Viperid Snake Venoms: Perspectives on Thromboinflammation', *Frontiers in Immunology*, 10 (2019) <https://doi.org/10.3389/fimmu.2019.02082>.

[18] John B. Harris and Tracey Scott-Davey, 'Secreted Phospholipases A2 of Snake Venoms: Effects on the Peripheral Neuromuscular System with Comments on the Role of Phospholipases A2 in Disorders of the CNS and Their Uses in Industry', *Toxins*, 5.12 (2013), 2533–71 <https://doi.org/10.3390/toxins5122533>.

49

Dexamethasone has shown itself useful in counteracting the development of COVID-19 symptoms. This drug inhibits PLA2 by blocking the synthesis of prostaglandins and leukotriene formation at the level of cyclo-oxygenase/PGE isomerase.[19] Moreover, **dexamethasone** blocks the synthesis of cytokines IL1, IL2, IL3, IL6, TNF-alpha, GM-CSF, interferon, epidermal growth factor (EGF, stimulated by PLA2 (cPLA2)), and the release of arachidonic acid (AA) by stopping the recruitment of Grb2 to the activated EGF receptor (EGF-R) through a transcription-independent mechanism (actinomycin-insensitive).[20]

As we have already mentioned, the PLA2 determines the release of fatty acids and the related production of lysophospholipids by mediating the hydrolysis of glycerophospholipids.

<Arachidonic acid (AA) is generated by membrane phospholipids through their activation. From arachidonic acid, by means of cycloxygenase-1 (COX-1), prostaglandins (PG) are generated, and by means of thromboxane synthetics, thromboxane A2 (TXA2) is generated. Prostaglandin E (PGE)

---

[19] M. Goppelt-Struebe, D. Wolter, and K. Resch, 'Glucocorticoids Inhibit Prostaglandin Synthesis Not Only at the Level of Phospholipase A2 but Also at the Level of Cyclo-Oxygenase/PGE Isomerase.', *British Journal of Pharmacology*, 98.4 (1989), 1287–95.

[20] Jamie D Croxtall, Qam Choudhury, and Rod J Flower, 'Glucocorticoids Act within Minutes to Inhibit Recruitment of Signalling Factors to Activated EGF Receptors through a Receptor-Dependent, Transcription-Independent Mechanism', *British Journal of Pharmacology*, 130.2 (2000), 289–98 <https://doi.org/10.1038/sj.bjp.0703272>.

causes both vasodilation and vasoconstriction, but in the pulmonary circle it determines only vasoconstriction. Prostaglandins E and F (PGE and PGF) increase the heart range. TXA2 is a molecule with high platelet aggregating power, vasoconstrict, capable of reducing renal blood flow and its filtration>.[21]

Dazoxiben and Pirmagrel block the enzyme thromboxane synthase. It increases the synthesis of prostaglandins through isomerase (PGD2, PGF2alfa, and PGE2) and prostacyclin synthase (PGI2, PGF1 alpha).[22] Inhibition of COX-1 leads to the lipoxygenase pathway growth and an increased leukotriene end-product volume (LB4, LC4, LD4, LE4, LF4).

<LTC4 and LTD4 are a thousand times more powerful than histamine, acting on the smooth muscles of the peripheral respiratory tract causing bronchoconstriction>.[23]

Toxins (PLA2 in particular), produced by infected bacteria, activate the arachidonic acid pathway. It means that we should avoid the therapeutic administration of cycloxygenase-1

---

[21] 'Goodman & Gilman's: The Pharmacological Basis of Therapeutics, 13e | AccessMedicine | McGraw-Hill Medical'.

[22] Fiddler, G. I. and P. Lumley, 'Preliminary Clinical Studies with Thromboxane Synthase Inhibitors and Thromboxane Receptor Blockers. A Review', *Circulation*, 81.1 Suppl (1990), 169-78; discussion 179-80.

[23] 'Goodman & Gilman's: The Pharmacological Basis of Therapeutics, 13e | AccessMedicine | McGraw-Hill Medical'.

inhibitors (anti-COX-1 NSAIDs, e.g. ibuprofen, nimesulide, paracetamol, etc.).

Antibiotics

Between the 14th and 21st day of bacterial and viral culture in vitro, we performed an antibiogram to see which antibiotic molecules prevented both viral replication and toxin production.[24] The data showed that azithromycin, metronidazole, and vancomycin extinguished viral replication and toxin generation in 3 days. In contrast, amoxicillin stopped viral replication but not the release of some new toxins. However, there were no conotoxins or phospholipases A2 amongst them. Other antibiotics helped in reducing viral replication. Wherein, some of them, such as levofloxacin, on the contrary - amplified it. After repeating these tests many times, we realised that bacteria have their own defence mechanism against the new pathogens. Unfortunately, the toxic proteins they produce while fighting the virus affect our target organs and receptors, determining the clinical picture of the COVID-19 patients.

---

[24] Petrillo and others. 'Increase of SARS-CoV-2 RNA Load in Faecal Samples Prompts for Rethinking of SARS-CoV-2 Biology and COVID-19 Epidemiology', 2020 <https://doi.org/10.5281/zenodo.4088208>

Stages of pathogenesis

There are two SARS-CoV-2 transmission pathway:
1.Fecal–oral
2.Respiratory

The virus can colonize the following mucous membranes:
1.Oral mucosa
2.Nasal and pharyngeal mucosa
3.Respiratory mucosa
4.Intestinal mucosa
5.Anal mucosa
6.Mucous membranes of the reproductive system

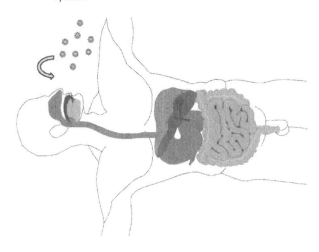

Figure 13: **Phase 1.** The virus attacks bacteria on the mucous membrane. Dr C. Brogna - Craniomed Group. All rights reserved.

55

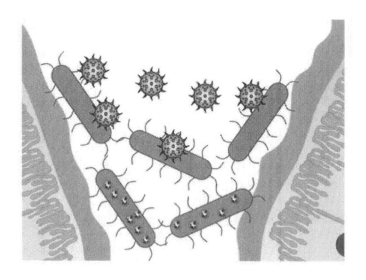

Figure 14: **Phase 2.** The bacteria produce a cascade of toxins. Dr C. Brogna - Craniomed Group. All rights reserved.

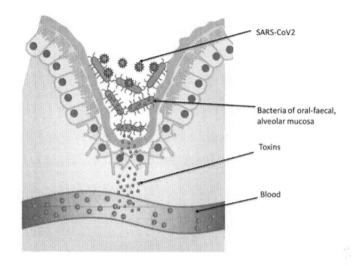

Figure 15: **Phase 3.** Produced toxins enter the circulatory system. Dr C. Brogna - Craniomed Group. All rights reserved.

57

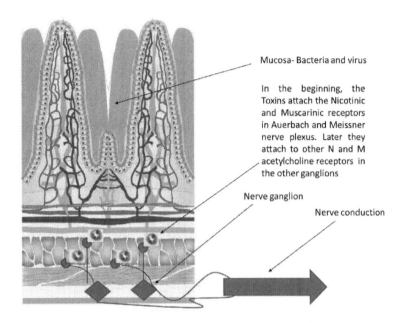

Mucosa- Bacteria and virus

In the beginning, the Toxins attach the Nicotinic and Muscarinic receptors in Auerbach and Meissner nerve plexus. Later they attach to other N and M acetylcholine receptors in the other ganglions

Nerve ganglion

Nerve conduction

Figure 16: **Phase 4.** Some toxins attack the enteric nervous system (Auerbach's and Meissner's plexuses; sympathetic and parasympathetic)[25] and all the ganglia of the autonomic nervous system. Dr C. Brogna - Craniomed Group. All rights reserved.

---

[25] Brogna and others.

Toxins bind to host molecules, such as acetylcholinesterase, thus enhancing the effects of acetylcholine on nicotinic and muscarinic receptors. Preganglionic neurons, both parasympathetic and sympathetic, are cholinergic, and ganglion transmission occurs thanks to nicotinic receptors (although excitatory muscarinic receptors are also present on postganglionic cells). Parasympathetic postganglionic neurons are cholinergic and act on muscarinic receptors present in the target organs. Sympathetic postganglionic neurons are essentially non-cholinergic, with rare exceptions in which they are cholinergic (e.g., sweat glands).

Note: The patients, who took azithromycin or amoxicillin combined with probiotics (Lactobacillus Reuteri and Bacillus clausii) at *time zero,* without taking any nonsteroidal anti-inflammatory drugs or cyclooxygenase-1 inhibitors (paracetamol), had a prompt recovery and mild initial symptoms.

PART 3

An observation or a mysterious discovery?

In the samples submitted for bacterial and viral culture, we can observe two strange phenomena that have never been described before:

1.   An **endoskeleton** of SARS-CoV-2 (Fig. 2, 17-22)
2.   Virion **fusion or scission**? (Fig. 18, 20-24)
The following images illustrate our discovery.

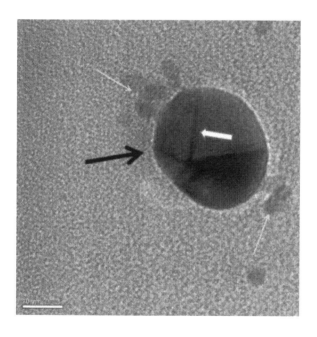

Figure 17: TEM image. SARS-CoV-2 in a faecal sample after the seven-day culture. You can see its "corona" (black arrow), the

61

proteins/toxins (thin arrows) around it, and the mysterious "endoskeleton" inside it (white arrow). Dr C. Brogna - Craniomed Group.

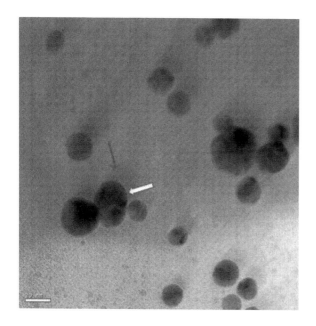

Figure 18: TEM image. SARS-CoV-2 in a faecal sample during the seven-day culture. You can see the virus (thin arrow) and its mysterious "endoskeleton" (white arrow). The virus particles and its "corona" are smaller (50-200 nm) than their usual size described in the scientific literature (0.1-0.3 μ). Dr C. Brogna- Craniomed Group.

63

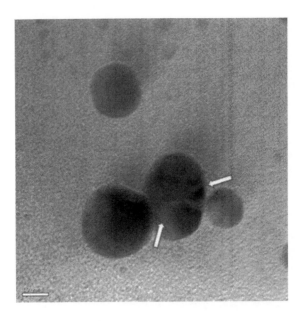

Figure 19: TEM image. SARS-CoV-2 in a faecal sample during the seven-day culture. An enlarged photo from Figure 18. You can see the mysterious "endoskeleton" (white arrows). The virus particles and its "corona" are smaller (50-200 nm) than their usual size described in the scientific literature (0.1-0.3 μ). Dr C. Brogna - Craniomed Group.

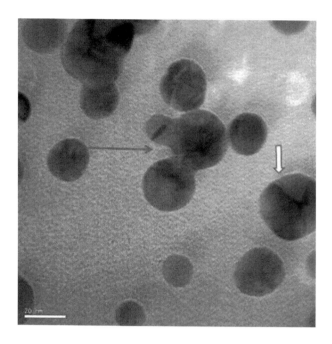

Figure 20: TEM image. SARS-CoV-2 in a faecal sample during the seven-day culture. You can see a strange "fusion" of the virions (long arrow). The virus particles and its "corona" are smaller (50-200 nm) than their usual size described in the scientific literature (0.1-0.3 μ). The white arrow indicates a mysterious "endoskeleton". Dr C. Brogna - Craniomed Group.

65

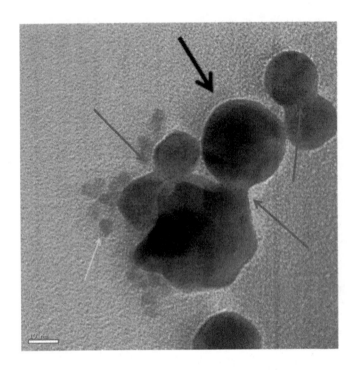

Figure 21: TEM image. SARS-CoV-2 in a faecal sample during the seven-day culture. You can see its "corona", the proteins/toxins (thin arrow) around it, and a strange "fusion" (or scission?) of the virions (long arrows). Dr C. Brogna - Craniomed Group.

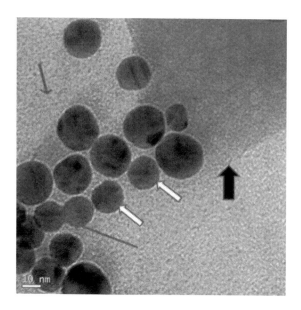

Figure 22: TEM image. SARS-CoV-2 and the bacterial cell walls in a faecal sample during the seven-day culture. You can see the virus (arrow) attacking the bacterium (big arrow) and its mysterious "endoskeleton" (white arrow). There is a strange "fusion" or agglomeration of the virions (long arrow). The virus particles and its "corona" are smaller (50-200 nm) than their usual size described in the scientific literature (0.1-0.3 μ). Dr C. Brogna - Craniomed Group. All rights reserved.

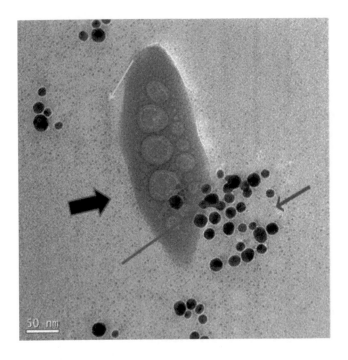

Figure 23: TEM image. A faecal sample during the seven-day culture. SARS-CoV-2 (arrow) is attacking the bacteria (big arrow). There is a strange "fusion" or agglomeration of the virions (long arrow). The virus particles and its "corona" are smaller (50-200 nm) than their usual size described in the scientific literature (0.1-0.3 μ). The thin arrow indicates the proteins/toxins. Dr C. Brogna - Craniomed Group. All rights reserved.

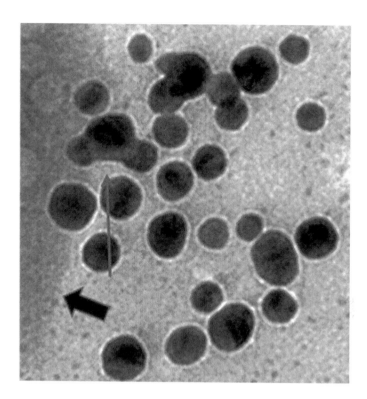

Figure 24: TEM image. SARS-CoV-2 and bacteria in a faecal sample during the seven-day culture. It is an enlarged photo from Figure 23. Dr C. Brogna - Craniomed Group.

Based on what has been observed so far, perhaps, we should evaluate the hypothesis that SARS-CoV-2 is not just a virus, but also something more complex.

Rises in neutrophil levels usually occur naturally due to bacterial pathogenesis. Could it possibly be a viral cDNA in an artificial plasmid, a hybrid with the face of coronavirus and the heart of a bacterium?

Considering the reduced virion size (50-200 nm), we could not help but wonder if it is a BAC (bacterial artificial chromosome) with a mantle consisting of coronavirus S proteins.

After carefully analysing all the evidence, obtained during the research phases, surely we cannot overlook the fact that SARS-CoV-2 is also **a bacteriophage.**

Considerations

For a long time, the researchers limited their curiosity. They observed pathogenic microorganisms and their pathogenicity, focused on understanding their connection with our cell surface receptors. The inhibition of such bonds was a basis for many treatments.

Only in a few exceptional cases, such as tetanus, botulism, and diphtheria, the specialists realized that the symptoms of the disease were related to the circulation of toxins.

The research field needs to make a qualitative leap forward and focus its attention on the entropy of the bacterial world. Yes, this is not a mistake: "entropy". In this never-ending scientific story, physicists are probably right.

Every energy-consuming system produces entropy. This mechanism involves multicellular beings and single-celled bacteria, as well.

Commensals, living in our body, produce protein-rich waste.

We are immunized towards these waste proteins from an early age, thanks to maternal antibodies and individual immune system.

The problem arises, when the bacteria react to a chemical (e.g., pollution) or biological insult (in case of SARS-CoV-2). As a result, they begin producing modified metabolic waste - completely new proteins unknown to our immune system, which cannot cope with it.

For this reason, a cure that prevents SARS-CoV-2 from binding with our cells and does not consider the nature of bacteriophage will not be sufficient.

We need to protect our friendly bacteria and find an antidote against the toxins they produce after viral aggression.

Bacteria can defend themselves, but we are not ready to dispose of the toxic waste they leave on the battlefield.

There is no sense in continuously disinfecting roads, public transport, and urban spaces, following the standard protocols. We risk paying a high price for ignoring the fact that the virus replicates in bacteria.

The observation that toxins are more active at low temperatures (spring, autumn, and winter) and less so during warm periods, does not explain thoroughly why the virus has particular seasonal trends.

Foremost, we need to remember, that we are talking about a bacteriophage (or maybe something different - BAC (bacterial artificial chromosome) - plasmid)[26], and as such it is ubiquitous.

It is a third big mistake to presume that SARS-CoV-2 does not contaminate the nature around us. It seems logical that a bacteriophage like this can infect sewage and wastewaters, and consequently everything downstream, starting with the agricultural sector and fisheries.

---

[26] Fernando Almazán, Carmen Galán, and Luis Enjuanes, 'Engineering Infectious CDNAs of Coronavirus as Bacterial Artificial Chromosomes', *Methods in Molecular Biology*, 454 (2008) <https://doi.org/10.1007/978-1-59745-181-9_20>.

Since we know that after being attacked by the virus bacteria start producing toxins, we can assume that vaccinated people may develop an increased risk of heart disease, accelerated blood clotting, and neurodegenerative lung diseases in the upcoming years.

We should probably expect countless mutations in the protein structure of SARS-CoV-2 bacteriophage, different after every replication cycle and every individual. Why? Because bacteria generate "editing" errors - they introduce new sequences, designed to help them cope with the future viral attack. The problem is that the infection will continue spreading all around the world. The bacteria of an immune individual will recognize the virus next time it approaches their host's body; however, it will not work for another person.[27]

[27]Rodolphe Barrangou and others, 'CRISPR Provides Acquired Resistance against Viruses in Prokaryotes', *Science (New York, N.Y.)* , 315.5819 (2007), 1709–12 <https://doi.org/10.1126/science.1138140>.

PART 4

Glossary

Acetylcholine (ACh) is a neurotransmitter in the central and peripheral nervous system. It binds to nicotinic or muscarinic receptors and mediates multiple functions: skeletal muscle contraction; nerve impulse transmission through synthetic pathways; and gland activity.

Acetylcholinesterase (AChE) is an enzyme that catalyses the breakdown of acetylcholine, inactivating it.

Amino acid is an organic molecule, a protein building block.

Antibiotic is a very complex chemical structure active against bacteria. It stops bacteria from reproducing (bacteriostat) or kills them (bactericide).

Antihypertensive is the drug that can reduce blood pressure.

Autonomic nervous system (ANS) is a part of the nervous system that regulates vegetative functions, i.e., those phenomena that we cannot control, such as the heartbeat, for example. It is divided into the sympathetic and parasympathetic nervous systems, which often produce the opposite effects. For example, the sympathetic system determines the pupil dilation (mydriasis) and parasympathetic system - its narrowing (myosis).

Bacterial editing is a natural defence mechanism of bacteria (CRISP). It allows them to generate errors/mutations in bacteriophages.

Bacteriophage, also known as phage, is a DNA or RNA virus that infects bacteria, inoculating its genetic material and replicating within them.

Bacterium is a single-celled organism, prokaryote, approximately 0.2 to 30 microns big. Its cell wall covers a cell membrane, containing the genetic material (unlike eukaryotic cell DNA, bacterial DNA is not encapsulated). A bacterium has an enzymatic system that allows them to produce energy and synthesise proteins, and thus replicate by splitting.

It can be lysogenic (i.e. remain integrated into the bacterium and replicate whenever the host bacterium replicates), lithic (i.e. replicate in the bacterium, literally inducing its destruction) or temperate (i.e. have a mixed behaviour based on dynamic balances).

Biochemistry is the branch of biology that studies chemical reactions within the living organisms.

Biology is a natural science that studies life and living organisms.

Blood clotting is a complex biological process of the formation of blood clots (necessary to control the bleeding when the vascular system is damaged) or thrombi (a pathological process that can provoke the vascular occlusion).

Bronchoconstriction is a condition in which the smooth muscles of the bronchi contract. The bronchial spasm causes severe breathing difficulties due to the reduced amount of air passing into the lungs.

Central nervous system (CNS) is a part of the nervous system consisting of the brain, protected by the skull, and the spinal cord within the vertebral canal.

Cholinergic activity is mediated by acetylcholine and, therefore, stimulates the parasympathetic autonomic nervous system. It controls functions of the various organs; for example, it regulates the constriction of the pupil, causing myosis, or reduces cardiac activity.

Cholinergic receptors (nicotinic (N) and muscarinic (M1, M2, M3 etc.)) are the receptors (proteins with "lock function") situated on various levels of the cell membranes. Molecules or small proteins (called ligands - proteins with "key function", such as acetylcholine) bind to these receptors allowing the perception of the nerve impulse.

Coronavirus is a family of RNA viruses that got its name from its appearance. Under a microscope, the spike protein resembles a solar corona.

Cycloxygenase-1 is an enzyme that accelerates the synthesis of prostaglandins.

Dexamethasone is a synthetic corticosteroid that has a strong anti-inflammatory and anti-allergic effect.

Dysgeusia is an alteration of the normal gustatory functioning.

Embolism is the blood vessel occlusion, caused by a foreign body (embolus). It can be a blood clot (thromboembolism), a bubble of air or another gas, fatty tissue and other unattached mass.

Endoskeleton (from ancient Greek ἔνδον - "within, inner" and σκελετός - "skeleton") is an internal support structure of an organism. The human skeletal system is an endoskeleton. The term is misused in image descriptions in order to illustrate a new phenomenon observed in SARS-CoV-2.

Enzyme is a protein substance capable of accelerating a specific chemical reaction without degrading.

Acetylcholinesterase, for example, accelerates the detachment of acetylcholine from the receptor to which it is bound. Otherwise, this process would be too slow. It could bring a number of functional and clinical implications.

Epidemiology is the branch of medicine that studies all the factors that determine the presence or absence of diseases. Epidemiological research helps us to understand how many people have a disease and if those numbers are changing.

Epithelial cells are a type of cell that forms the epithelial tissue. They are involved in various processes: the lining of the body surfaces (skin and mucous membranes); secretion (glands); transportation and absorption (intestinal mucous membranes).

Eukaryotic cells (from ancient Greek ευ - "well, completely" and κάρυον – "nucleus") are the most advanced cells. The human body consists of such cells. Their main feature is that the genetic material (DNA) is enclosed in the nucleus, which separates it from the cytoplasm (the semi-liquid contents of the cell).

Genome is all genetic information - DNA (or, in some viruses - RNA) - contained in a cell or organism.

Gut flora or gut microbiota is a set of bacteria that colonise the intestines and perform several functions. It autoregulates itself, keeps a certain balance between different species, preventing the growth of potentially harmful bacteria, that can cause pathological conditions.

Hyposmia is a reduced olfactory sensitivity.

Mass spectrometry is a technique that uses static or oscillating magnetic fields to identify substances and compounds. Ion mixtures (atoms or groups of charged atoms) are separated according to their mass-to-charge ratio. An analytical approach is usually employed in combination with separation techniques, such as high-performance liquid chromatography (HPLC).

Metabolism is the set of chemical processes occurring within a living cell or organism necessary to maintain life. These enzyme-accelerated (catalysed) reactions allow organisms to grow and reproduce, maintain their structures, and generate the stress response.

Microbiology is the branch of biology that studies microorganisms. Biologists use optical microscopes to observe living beings (eukaryotes, prokaryotes, and viruses) that are too small to see with the naked eye.

Nerve cell, also known as neuron, is a fundamental component of the nervous tissue. It transmits the electrical signals carrying information (perception of pain or muscular contraction).

Neurotoxin is a toxin that acts on the cells of the nervous system.

Neurotransmitter is a substance that allows transmitting the nerve impulses (and all the attached information) from one neuron to another.

Nucleic acids are organic chemical compounds essential to all known forms of life (including viruses). The two main classes of nucleic acids are deoxyribonucleic acid (DNA) and ribonucleic acid (RNA).

DNA codes genetic information contained in cells. RNA translates and transfers the information contained in DNA in order to begin protein synthesis and cell replication.

Nucleotide is an organic compound, the building block of nucleic acids (DNA or RNA).

Olfactory bulb is the first olfactory pulse processing station, located between the nasal cavities and the base of the skull.

Peripheral nervous system (PNS) is a part of the nervous system containing bundles of nerve fibres that connect the central nervous system to the different organs (heart, muscles, sense organs, glands, etc.).

Plasmid is a small circular strand of DNA present within bacteria that performs various non-essential functions and endows the cell with special, sometimes unique properties. Plasmids can move between cells.

Platelet is a corpuscular element of the blood (it is not a cell, but a cell fragment). Platelets assist blood clotting process by aggregating in a specific area (platelet aggregation).

Probiotics are the beneficial microorganisms that live in the digestive system and maintain normal microflora in it. Probiotics are a result of lactic fermentation (Lactobacillus acidophilus, for example). They produce a positive effect on the host's organism (human or another mammal) and shield it from pathogenic organisms.

Prokaryotic cell (from ancient Greek πρό - "before" and κάρυον - "nucleus") is a "primitive" cell that does not have a formed nucleus. Most prokaryotes are bacteria.

Prostaglandin is a molecule that mediates many biochemical processes, including inflammation, pain sensitivity, fever, etc.

Protein is a biological macromolecule that consists of one or more chains of amino acids.

Protein synthesis is a biochemical process through which the genetic information contained in DNA is converted into proteins, performing a wide range of functions in the cell.

SARS-CoV-2 is a virus belonging to the Betacoronavirus family, responsible for acute respiratory stress syndrome.

SEM is a scanning electron microscope. It uses a beam of light as an emission source and gives a 3D image. The resolution limit of electron microscope is about 0.2nm.

Symptom is a subjective description of the patient's altered state of health. As opposed to a symptom, a sign is objective evidence of disease. For example, in the case of a puncture wound - pain is a symptom and bleeding is a sign.

TEM is a transmission electron microscope. It uses a vacuum electron beam that passes through the specimen. The resolution of a TEM is about 0.2 nm.

Toxin is a biological substance (generally a protein composed of a relatively small number of amino acids - oligopeptide) produced by microbes (i.e., bacteria, fungi), plants (phytotoxins) or animals (zootoxins). Even small doses of toxins can produce harmful effects on living beings. Infectious diseases caused by pathogenic organisms that produce toxins are called "toxinfections". Patients with such diseases present the signs of poisoning and tend to have severe deterioration of the general condition.

Vero Cell is a synthetic cell deriving from the kidney of a monkey. It is used to perform cell cultures.

Virus is an organism of submicroscopic size and non-cellular nature (unlike bacteria, which are prokaryotic cells), consisting mostly of the nucleic acid (DNA or RNA) coated and protected by envelope protein, called "capsid". Some of the capsid proteins allow the virus to adhere to the target cell. Since the viruses do not have an enzyme system necessary for energy production and protein synthesis (fundamental processes for their replication and, therefore, survival), viruses are forced to use other cells (eukaryotes, such as human cells, or prokaryotes, such as bacterial cells), i.e., the infected host cells.

Criticism of science

Dear researcher, if you are an academic or not, I think you have already understood that I do not consider the expert opinions too important and that I dare to contradict them.

In 1517, Martin Luther formulated 95 theses and waited for the bishops to change their orientation for two years, but everything was in vain. Afterwards, he decided to address ordinary people and translate the New Testament from Latin to German. This way, the knowledge became available to everyone; people could finally read it.

Christopher Columbus set sail from Palos de la Frontera on 3rd August 1492 and arrived in present-day El Salvador on 12th October of the same year. He faced a journey with many sailors and three caravels, hoping to find India. Despite possible mutiny and various navigation difficulties, after 90 days, he arrived in the new lands. The Europeans had to wait for a long time before taking the same paths and making their own discoveries.

Other experts in their field are not always determined enough. They are not ready to overcome the difficulties that arise during the research process. Often, the desire to criticise kills the spirit of cohesion. We need to think outside the box in order to face the great challenges, like a pandemic.

Making breakthrough attempts without considering **that SARS-Cov-2 is, primarily, a bacteriophage** (or perhaps something even more complex), is like trying to see the other 75 moons of Jupiter using the telescope manufactured by Galileo Galilei.

That is why I am telling you: "Repeat my experiments first, and then, come look for me on one of the 79 moons orbiting Jupiter."

Acknowledgements

Before all else, I would like to thank Dr Gianluca Ciammetti, head of the department of otolaryngology at F. Veneziale Hospital Isernia, who has been supporting the research from the very beginning.

I would never have finished this work without my fellow student and a co-author of this study - Dr Francesco Lauritano. In the moment of difficulty, I found a great friend.

A big thank you goes to Dr Domenico Bisaccia, a friend and a fellow student. Together with him, we discovered the replication of SARS-CoV-2 in bacteria.

I am very thankful to my friend Dr Giuliano Marino, Marsan Consulting, and all their friends.

With great esteem and affection, I thank Dr Francesco Marino, Dr Mirko Colella, Giancarlo Brogna, Giovanni Lombardi, and Gaetano Petrillo.

This journey would not have been possible without the dedicated support of Prof Ornella Piazza from the department of anesthesiology at the University of Salerno. She was the first person to hear about my discovery.

My friends, Dr Gennaro Iapicca, Atty Luigi Bergamino, and their families helped us a great deal during the experimentation phase.

Immense gratitude goes to my friend Dr Mauro Petrillo for helping me with the research.

The photos present in this work are property of Craniomed Group Srl.

Finally, I would like to express the most profound appreciation to Dr Simone Cristoni, one of the best experts in proteomics I have ever known. Without his valuable help, we would never have found toxins produced by bacteria in the plasma and urine of COVID-19 patients.

Most importantly, from the bottom of my heart, I thank the Creator.

He exists: הבורא קיים

SARS-CoV-2 in all its aspects. The unpublished photos, illustrating its mysterious nature, the way it replicates in bacteria, and the toxin synthesis. The incredible action of the neurotoxins that are killing so many people. This and much more about the interaction of the virus and bacteria in our body.

Supplementary data 1

Mass spectrometry analysis of protein

The following images represent some of the protein/toxin spectra found in plasma and urine of COVID-19 patients after performing faecal bacteria culture.

Mass spectrometry is an analytical technique that uses static or oscillating magnetic fields to identify unknown substances. Ion mixtures (atoms or groups of charged atoms) are separated according to their mass-to-charge ratio. An analytical approach is usually employed in combination with separation techniques, such as high-performance liquid chromatography (HPLC).

The mass spectra describe the discovered sequence of amino acids/toxins within a protein.

For more information, see "*C. Brogna and others, 'Detection of Toxin-like Peptides in Plasma and Urine Samples from COVID-19 Patients', 2020 <https://doi.org/10.5281/zenodo.413934>1*".

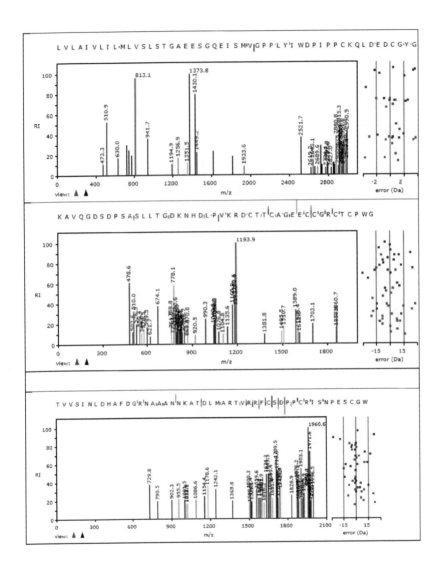

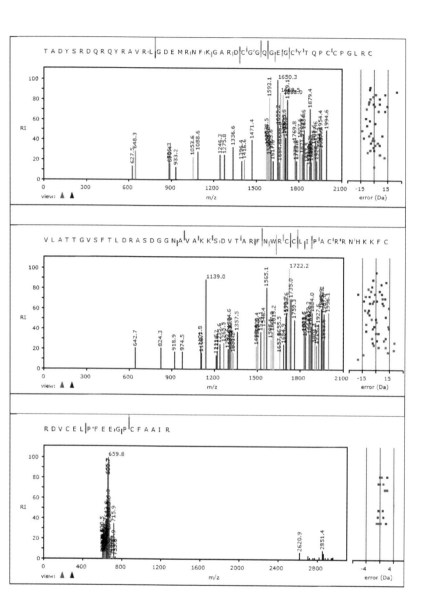

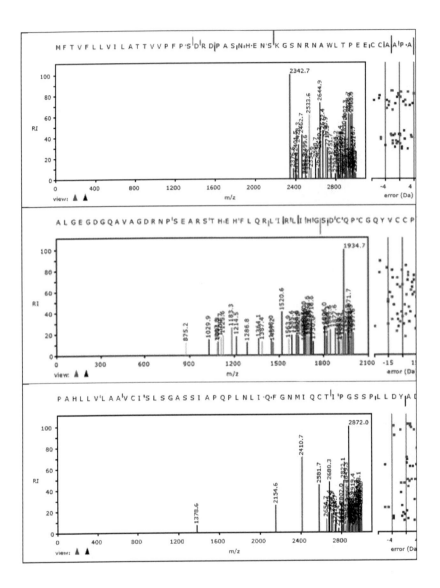

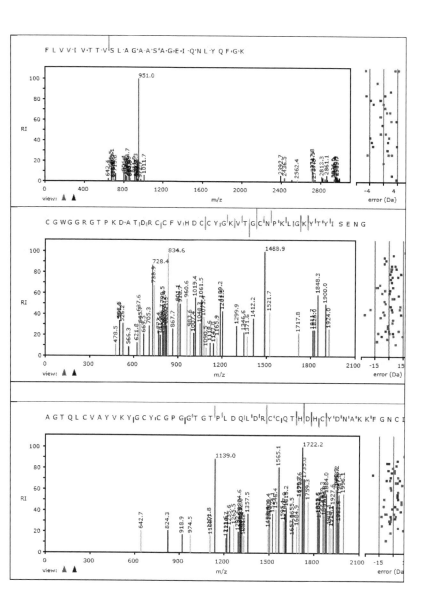

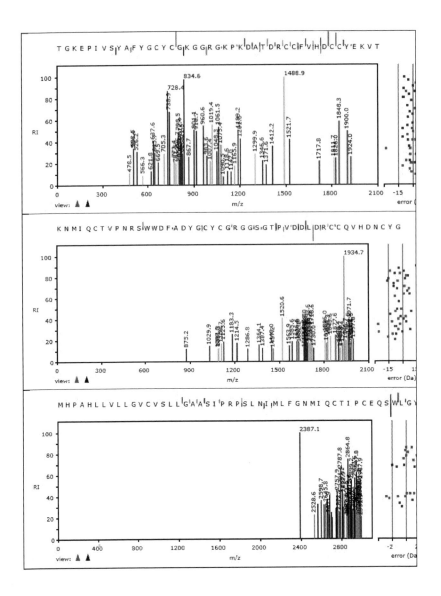

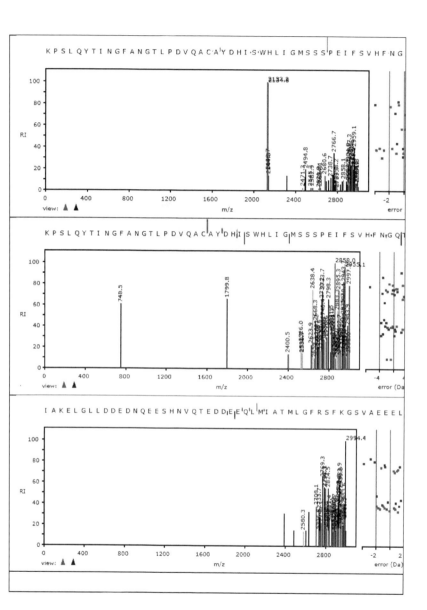

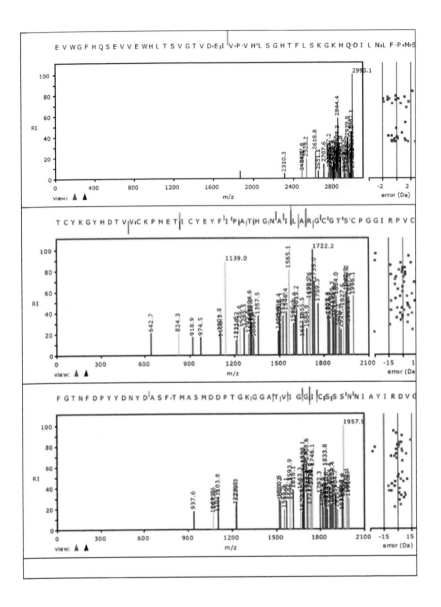

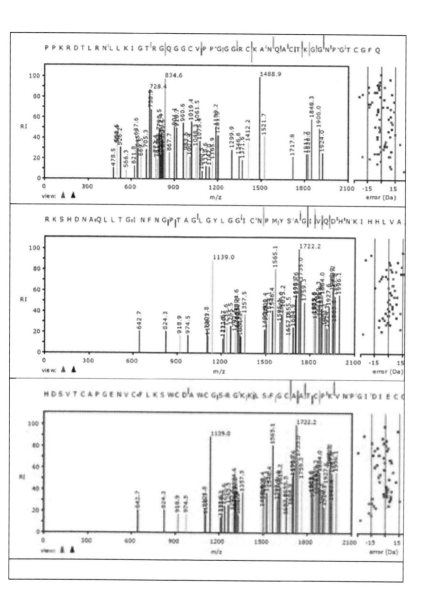

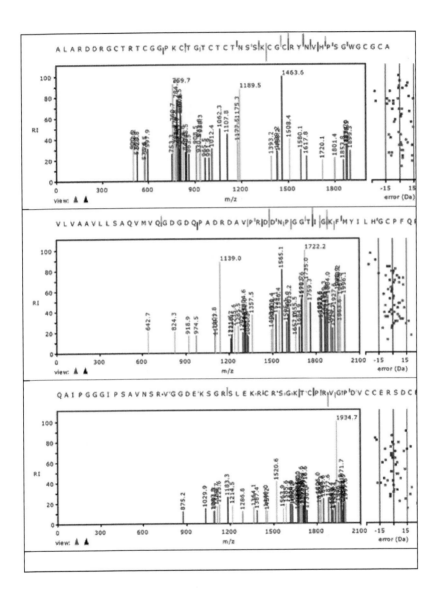

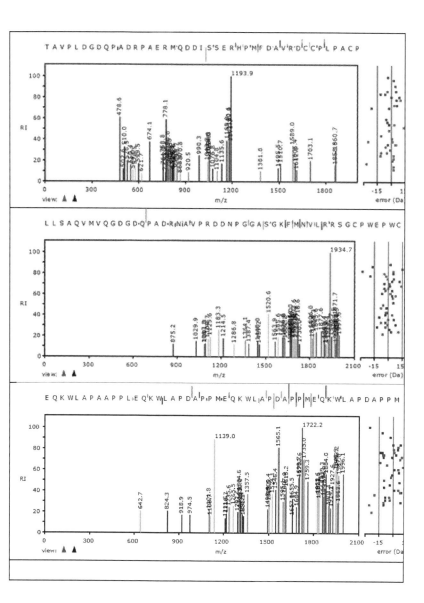

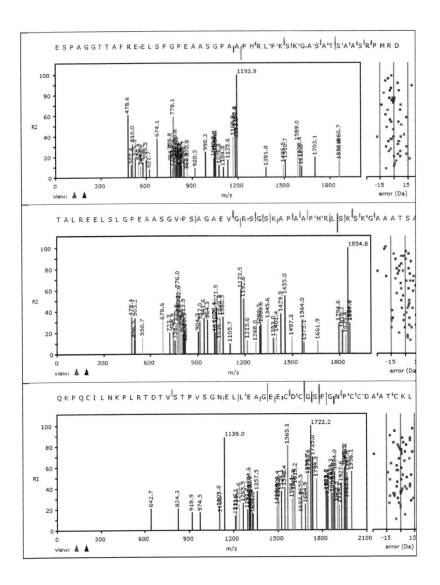

Supplementary data 2

The protein, similar to conotoxin.

The following images represent a conotoxin-like toxin/protein found in a COVID-19 patient.
The molecule is present several times in plasma and each time has some amino acid variants.
This event helped us understand that there were bacteria involved in the genesis of these toxins.

log(e) ▲	log(I)	%/%	#	total	Mr	Accession
-24.7	6.49	89/100+	2	2	8.9	sp|P0C8U9|CA15_CONPL gpmDB | psyt | snap [1/0] protein peptide Alpha-conotoxin-like Pu1.5; Flags: Precursor;
-17.8	6.00	54/100+	2	2	8.7	sp|Q9BPC3|O267_CONVE gpmDB | psyt | snap [1/0] homo (1/1) protein peptide Conotoxin VnMEKL-012; Flags: Precursor;
-16.6	6.20	62/100+	2	2	6.5	sp|P58809|CTAX_CONMR gpmDB | psyt | snap [1/0] protein peptide Chi-conotoxin CMrX; Conotoxin CMrX; Conotoxin Mr1.6, Lambda-conotoxin CMrX; Flags: Precursor;
-11.1	5.82	22/49	1	1	8.5	sp|D6C4M3|CU96_CONCL gpmDB | psyt | snap [1/0] protein peptide Conotoxin Cl9.6; Flags: Precursor;
-9.1	5.57	39/76	1	1	7.9	sp|B3FIA5|CVFA_CONVR gpmDB | psyt | snap [1/0] protein peptide Conotoxin Vil5a; Vil5.1; Flags: Precursor;
-6.4	5.30	34/51	1	1	8.5	sp|Q3YEG4|O1641_CONMI gpmDB | psyt | snap [1/0] homo (1/1) protein peptide Conotoxin MiK41; Flags: Precursor;
-5.9	5.32	38/48	1	1	7.4	sp|P0C667|CT52_CONCB gpmDB | psyt | snap [1/0] protein peptide Conotoxin Ca5.2 (ECO:0000303|PubMed:17933431); Flags: Precursor;
-5.2	6.37	78/100+	1	1	2.9	sp|P0C652|CLEA_CONCF gpmDB | psyt | snap [1/0] protein peptide Kappa-conotoxin-like as14a;
-4.9	5.61	28/40	1	1	8.3	sp|D2Y169|CU51C_CONCL gpmDB | psyt | snap [1/0] protein peptide Contains: Conotoxin Ca5a L3 {ECO:0000303|PubMed:21172372}; Contains: Conotoxin Ca5.1 {ECO:0000303|PubMed:21172372}; Flags: Precursor;
-2.2	6.32	22/23	1	2	8.6	sp|D2Y488|VKT1A_CONCL gpmDB | psyt | snap [1/0] homo (3/3) protein peptide Kunitz-type serine protease inhibitor conotoxin Cal9.1a; Flags: Precursor;
-2.0	5.68	25/31	1	1	7.4	sp|A0A2I6EDL6|CM38_CONRE gpmDB | psyt | snap [1/0] protein peptide Conotoxin reg3.8 {ECO:0000303|PubMed:29283511}; Rg3.8 {ECO:0000312|EMBL:AUI88066.1}; Flags: Precursor;
-1.9	5.43	28/49	1	1	6.9	sp|Q9BP53|CT0C5_CONVE gpmDB | psyt | snap [1/0] protein peptide Conotoxin VnMLCL-031; Flags: Precursor;

102

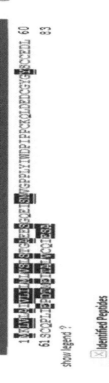

(validate)

show legend ?

☒ Identified Peptides

103

spectrum	log(e)	log(I)	m+h	delta	ζ	sequence	n
218.1	-6.9	5.28	8311.004	2.562	3/3	[¹]KLVLAIVLI LMLVSLSTGA EESGQEISMV GPPLYIWDPI PPCKQLDEDC GYGYSCCEDL SCQPLIEPDT MEITAL [⁷⁸]vcqi	(0)
923.1	-7.3	5.21	8471.071	2.087	3/3	[¹] MKLVLAIVLI LMLVSLSTGA EESGQEISMV GPPLYIWDPI PPCKQLDEDC GYGYSCCEDL SCQPLIEPDT MEITALVIC [⁷⁸]qies	(0)
921.1	-7.7	5.30	8883.266	2.802	3/3	[¹]KLVLAIVLI LMLVSLSTGA EESGQEISMV GPPLYIWDPI PPCKQLDEDC GYGYSCCEDL SCQPLIEPDT MEITALVCQI E [⁸¹,]sa]	(0)
974.1	-8.5	5.22	8495.088	-0.560	3/3	[mk²]LVLAIVLILM LVSLSTGAEE SGQEISMVGP PLYIWDPIPP CKQLDEDCGY GYSCCEDLSC QPLIEPDTME ITALVCQI [⁸⁰]esa]	(0)
602.1	-5.6	5.29	8453.078	-1.762	3/3	[mk²]LVLAIVLILM LVSLSTGAEE SGQEISMVGP PLYIWDPIPP CKQLDEDCGY GYSCCEDLSC QPLIEPDTME ITALVCQI [⁸⁰]esa]	(0)
1106.1	-11.9	5.43	8692.153	-1.260	3/3	[mk³]LVLAIVLILM LVSLSTGAEE SGQEISMVGP PLYIWDPIPP CKQLDEDCGY GYSCCEDLSC QPLIEPDTME ITALVCQIES A [⁸³]	(0)
1041.1	-8.5	5.28	8813.185	-0.167	3/3	[mk³]LVLAIVLILM LVSLSTGAEE SGQEISMVGP PLYIWDPIPP CKQLDEDCGY GYSCCEDLSC QPLIEPDTME ITALVCQIES A [⁸³]	(0)
1041.2	-8.5	5.28	8813.185	-0.167	3/3	[mk³]LVLAIVLILM LVSLSTGAEE SGQEISMVGP PLYIWDPIPP CKQLDEDCGY GYSCCEDLSC QPLIEPDTME ITALVCQIES A [⁸³]	(0)
404.1	-8.4	5.30	8696.181	1.778	3/3	[mk³]LVLAIVLILM LVSLSTGAEE SGQEISMVGP PLYIWDPIPP CKQLDEDCGY GYSCCEDLSC QPLIEPDTME ITALVCQIES A [⁸³]	(0)
296.1	-8.4	5.24	8754.205	1.790	3/3	[mk³]LVLAIVLILM LVSLSTGAEE SGQEISMVGP PLYIWDPIPP CKQLDEDCGY GYSCCEDLSC QPLIEPDTME ITALVCQIES A [⁸³]	(0)
296.2	-8.4	5.24	8754.169	1.827	3/3	[mk³]LVLAIVLILM LVSLSTGAEE SGQEISMVGP PLYIWDPIPP CKQLDEDCGY GYSCCEDLSC QPLIEPDTME ITALVCQIES A [⁸³]	(0)
296.3	-8.4	5.24	8754.169	1.827	3/3	[mk³]LVLAIVLILM LVSLSTGAEE SGQEISMVGP PLYIWDPIPP CKQLDEDCGY GYSCCEDLSC QPLIEPDTME ITALVCQIES A [⁸³]	(0)
296.4	-8.4	5.24	8754.205	1.790	3/3	[mk³]LVLAIVLILM LVSLSTGAEE SGQEISMVGP PLYIWDPIPP CKQLDEDCGY GYSCCEDLSC QPLIEPDTME ITALVCQIES A [⁸³]	(0)
296.5	-8.4	5.24	8754.205	1.790	3/3	[mk³]LVLAIVLILM LVSLSTGAEE SGQEISMVGP PLYIWDPIPP CKQLDEDCGY GYSCCEDLSC QPLIEPDTME ITALVCQIES A [⁸³]	(0)
504.1	-8.0	5.26	8797.226	3.917	3/3	[mk³]LVLAIVLILM LVSLSTGAEE SGQEISMVGP PLYIWDPIPP CKQLDEDCGY GYSCCEDLSC QPLIEPDTME ITALVCQIES A [⁸³]	(0)
504.2	-8.0	5.26	8797.226	3.917	3/3	[mk³]LVLAIVLILM LVSLSTGAEE SGQEISMVGP PLYIWDPIPP CKQLDEDCGY GYSCCEDLSC QPLIEPDTME ITALVCQIES A [⁸³]	(0)

104

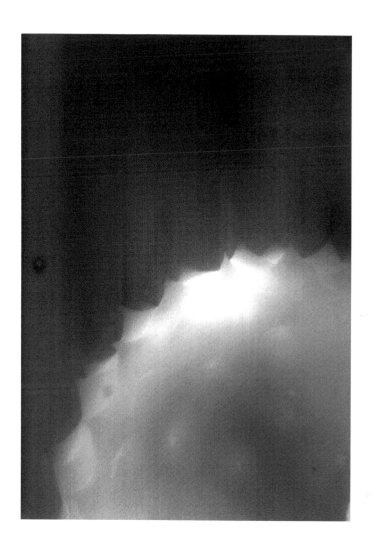

Printed in Great Britain
by Amazon

41243172R00059